THE ALL (ACUTE LYMPHOBLASTIC LEUKEMIA) HANDBOOK

A Guide for Parents and Young Warriors

Dr. Bhratri Bhushan MD, DM

Copyright © 2024 Dr. Bhratri Bhushan

Copyright © 2024 by Dr. Bhratri Bhushan

All rights reserved. No part of this publication may be reproduced, distributed, or transmitted in any form or by any means, including photocopying, recording, or other electronic or mechanical methods, without the prior written permission of the publisher, except in the case of brief quotations embodied in critical reviews and certain other noncommercial uses permitted by copyright law.

For permission requests, write to the publisher, addressed "Attention: Permissions Coordinator," at the address:

A30, Ananta institute of medical sciences,
Rajsamand, Rajasthan, India 313202
Email: www.bhratri@gmail.com

This work is provided "as is," and the author and the publisher disclaim any and all warranties, express or implied, including any warranties as to accuracy, comprehensiveness, or currency of the content of this work.

To the maximum extent permitted under applicable law, no responsibility is assumed by the publisher for any injury and/or damage to persons or property as a matter of products liability, negligence law or otherwise, or from any reference to or use by any person of this work.

CONTENTS

Title Page
Copyright
Preface
What is acute lymphoblastic leukemia?   1
What causes ALL to develop?   3
What are the symptoms of ALL?   4
What tests and procedures are used to diagnose ALL?   6
Describe a typical workup for ALL   10
Genetic abnormalities and molecular subtypes of ALL   12
Prognostic factors and risk stratification   19
What are the key treatment phases and therapeutic agents to consider in managing ALL?   24
How can extramedullary disease be prevented and treated in ALL?   29
What is the role of hematopoietic cell transplantation (HCT) in the treatment of ALL?   30

What is the role of targeted therapies in the treatment of ALL?   32

What are the key treatment considerations for adolescent and young adult (AYA) patients with ALL?   34

What are the treatment challenges and considerations for vulnerable populations in ALL?   36

How is minimal residual disease (MRD) used to guide treatment decisions in ALL?   38

How is BCR::ABL1-negative or BCR::ABL1-like B-ALL managed?   42

How is BCR::ABL1-positive B-ALL managed?   55

Management of T-ALL   61

Management of Infant ALL   66

Evaluation and Treatment of Extramedullary Disease   70

Response Assessment and Surveillance   73

Supportive Care for Pediatric Patients with ALL   77

What is the typical experience of a patient with ALL and their family during the course of diagnosis   82

What lifestyle advice, food preferences, and precautions should be followed by patients undergoing A   89

What are the common complications of ALL treatment, and how can families effectively manage them?   96

| Letter to a reader | 104 |
| About The Author | 107 |

PREFACE

Revised and updated for 2025.

Acute Lymphoblastic Leukemia (ALL) is one of the most challenging types of leukemia, primarily affecting children and young adults worldwide. With remarkable advancements in diagnostic methods, risk stratification, and treatment protocols, the management of ALL has transformed significantly, offering better outcomes and hope for patients and their families.

In this book, we will explore the complexities of ALL, helping you gain a deeper understanding of this intricate disease. Learning that your child or a loved one has been diagnosed with ALL can be an overwhelming experience. It may seem daunting to invest time in understanding the biology and treatment of ALL during such a difficult period, but trust me—it is a crucial step in navigating this journey with confidence.

Modern medicine, particularly in oncology, has embraced the concept of "shared" decision-making.

This approach ensures that the treating team collaborates closely with families, empowering them to make informed choices together. As a parent, caregiver, or patient, your understanding of ALL is vital to this process. Knowledge not only provides clarity but also strengthens your ability to advocate for the best care.

The goal of this book is not to overwhelm you with technical jargon or exhaustive details but to provide clear, practical, and relevant information tailored to your needs. It is structured in an interactive format —questions and answers—designed to address common concerns and key topics based on my years of conversations with patients and their families.

This book is here to serve as a supportive companion, equipping you with the understanding and confidence needed to face ALL with resilience and hope. Together, let us navigate this challenging yet hopeful journey toward healing.

WHAT IS ACUTE LYMPHOBLASTIC LEUKEMIA?

Acute lymphoblastic leukemia is a type of **blood cancer** where **immature** white blood cells, called **lymphoblasts**, grow uncontrollably in the bone marrow, peripheral blood, and other organs. These abnormal cells crowd out healthy blood cells, causing problems like infections, anemia, and bleeding.

ALL can happen at any age, but it's most common in children, making up about 75% to 80% of childhood leukemia cases. It's less common in adults, accounting for about 20% of adult leukemias. While treatment has greatly improved over the years—especially for children, with survival rates reaching nearly 90%—the outcomes for adults are less favorable, with cure rates of about 20–40%. On the other hand, the survival rates for infant ALL (<1 year of age) have not seen any improvement with long term survival rate of nearly 60%.

Some facts about ALL:
1. ALL is the most common pediatric malignancy.
2. In the U.S., on average, for every 100,000 people in the population, approximately 1.38 new cases of ALL are diagnosed annually.

3. In the United States, each year there are approximately 7000 new cases and 1500 deaths due to ALL.
4. The median age of diagnosis for ALL is 15 years.

For the purpose of this book, the term **"pediatric"** in the context of ALL refers to patients **aged 18 years or younger** and, in certain cases, adolescent and young adult (AYA) patients older than 18 years who are treated in pediatric oncology settings. This definition acknowledges the variability in clinical practice, where **AYA patients**—commonly considered those —may receive treatment following pediatric protocols depending on institutional practices and referral patterns.

WHAT CAUSES ALL TO DEVELOP?

The **etiology** of a disease refers to the study of its causes or origins. In the case of acute lymphoblastic leukemia, the exact cause is often **unknown**, but several factors may contribute to an increased risk of developing the disease:

- Radiation exposure: High doses of radiation or prior radiation therapy for other cancers can raise the risk of ALL.
- Chemical exposure: Prolonged exposure to toxic chemicals like benzene is linked to a higher risk of ALL.
- Genetic disorders: Conditions such as Down syndrome, Fanconi anemia, neurofibromatosis, Klinefelter syndrome, Schwachman-Diamond syndrome, Bloom syndrome, Li-Fraumeni syndrome, and ataxia telangiectasia are associated with a higher likelihood of developing ALL.
- Age: The incidence of ALL is highest among children and adolescents under 15 years of age.
- Sex: Males are more frequently affected by ALL than females.
- Race/ethnicity: In the United States, ALL is more prevalent among Hispanics and whites.
- Viral infections: Certain viral infections, such as Epstein-Barr virus or human T-cell leukemia virus, can elevate the risk of ALL.

WHAT ARE THE SYMPTOMS OF ALL?

The clinical manifestations of ALL typically develop over a short period of time. The disease progresses rapidly, and the symptoms can become noticeable within days to weeks after the onset of abnormal cell proliferation.

The symptoms of ALL can vary depending on the extent of disease progression and the individual patient, but they typically include common signs of bone marrow dysfunction, such as fatigue, weakness, fever, frequent infections, and easy bruising or bleeding. Patients may also experience pale skin, shortness of breath, and an unexplained loss of appetite or weight. Swelling in the abdomen, chest, or lymph nodes can occur due to the accumulation of leukemia cells in these areas. The presence of lymphadenopathy, splenomegaly, and/or hepatomegaly on physical examination may be found in approximately 20% of patients. Bone or joint pain is another common symptom, as leukemia cells can infiltrate the bones. Among children, pain in the extremities or joints may be the only presenting symptom.

In some cases, rare symptoms can arise as well. These include persistent headaches, vomiting, and blurred vision, which may indicate central nervous system involvement. Chin numbness or facial palsy may result from cranial nerve or CNS involvement. Seizures can occasionally occur if leukemia cells spread to the brain. Unusual bleeding, such as nosebleeds, gum bleeding, or red spots on the skin (petechiae), can also be signs of the disease. In very rare instances, ALL may present with skin rashes, and less commonly, testicular enlargement in males. These symptoms are often due to the infiltration of leukemia cells in the respective organs.

In some cases, ALL can be asymptomatic at the time of presentation, particularly in the very early stages of the disease. However, this is relatively rare, as most patients eventually develop noticeable symptoms due to the rapid progression of the disease.

When ALL does present asymptomatically, it is often detected during routine blood tests, such as a complete blood count (CBC), which may show abnormal levels of white blood cells, anemia, or thrombocytopenia (low platelets). In these cases, the patient may have no obvious signs of the disease, but abnormal lab results prompt further investigation. However, the majority of patients with ALL do present with some combination of the common symptoms, which generally lead to seeking medical attention.

WHAT TESTS AND PROCEDURES ARE USED TO DIAGNOSE ALL?

To diagnose acute lymphoblastic leukemia, doctors typically need to find at least 20% lymphoblasts (immature white blood cells) in the bone marrow, which is determined through a review of bone marrow samples. In some treatment protocols, a higher threshold of 25% blasts is used to define leukemia. If fewer than 20% blasts are found, the diagnosis of ALL is unlikely.

If bone marrow samples cannot be obtained, doctors may look at blood samples instead, but only if there is a significant amount of leukemia cells in the blood. In such cases, a common guideline is that there should be at least 1000 lymphoblasts per microliter of blood or 20% of the blood cells should be lymphoblasts.

The World Health Organization (WHO) classifies ALL and lymphoblastic lymphoma (LL) as the same disease, with the difference being that LL is usually confined to lymph nodes or other sites, with minimal involvement of the blood or bone marrow. If the disease is found mainly in a mass or lymph nodes with fewer than 20% lymphoblasts in the marrow, it is considered lymphoblastic lymphoma. However, the disease is treated like ALL, and treatment should be carried out at a specialized center experienced in managing both ALL and LL.

Hematopathology evaluations for diagnosing ALL should involve a detailed examination of the malignant lymphocytes. This includes looking at slides stained with Wright-Giemsa and core biopsy or clot sections stained with hematoxylin and eosin to assess the cell's appearance under a microscope. Additionally, comprehensive immunophenotyping using flow cytometry is essential to identify the specific types of cells involved.

A baseline characterization of the leukemic clone(s) should also be performed through flow cytometry or molecular testing, such as analyzing immunoglobulin (Ig) or T-cell receptor (TCR) gene rearrangements. This helps in identifying the specific genetic features of the leukemia and is important for monitoring the disease, particularly for detecting minimal residual disease (MRD) during and after treatment.

Immunophenotyping is an important process for classifying acute lymphoblastic leukemia by analyzing the surface markers present on the lymphocytes. It is done using a technique called flow cytometry. There are two main types of ALL based on the immunophenotype: precursor B-cell ALL and T-cell ALL.

- Precursor B-cell ALL (B-ALL) accounts for about 80% of cases in children and 75% in adults. In B-ALL, the surface markers on the lymphocytes vary depending on the stage of B-cell development. Early precursor B-cell ALL is characterized by specific markers, such as the presence of terminal deoxynucleotidyl transferase (TdT), and the absence of others like CD10. The presence or absence of certain markers can also provide information about prognosis, such as the CD10 negativity being linked to a poor prognosis in cases with KMT2A gene rearrangements. Pre-B-cell ALL typically expresses markers like CD10, CD19, and CD22, and can show CD20 positivity in about 50% of cases, especially in children aged 1-10 years. Some genetic alterations, such as those involving the CRLF2 gene, can also be identified in pediatric cases.

- T-cell ALL represents around 10-15% of cases in children and 25% in adults. T-ALL is marked by the presence of cytoplasmic CD3 or cell surface CD3 and can have variable expression of markers like CD1a, CD2, CD5, and CD7, along with TdT expression. One specific subtype of T-ALL is early T-cell precursor (ETP) ALL, which is characterized by a lack of CD1a and CD8, weak expression of CD5, and the presence of markers typical of myeloid or stem cells, like CD34 and CD117. Though initially associated with poor outcomes, modern treatments have shown improved survival rates for ETP ALL patients.

In addition to these subtypes, ALL can sometimes present as mixed phenotype acute leukemia (MPAL), which features characteristics of both ALL and acute myeloid leukemia (AML). This condition may present with two distinct populations of leukemia cells or with a single population expressing markers from both B- or T-cell ALL and myeloid markers, such as CD13 or CD33. The expression of these myeloid markers does not exclude ALL and is not necessarily a sign of worse prognosis.

Immunophenotyping is also used to identify acute leukemias of ambiguous lineage (ALALs), such as MPALs, which may require comprehensive testing to accurately classify the leukemia and guide treatment decisions. The updated 2022 WHO classification has refined these criteria, adding new subtypes of ALAL based on genetic rearrangements, such as ZNF384 and BCL11B.

This detailed evaluation helps in identifying the specific type of ALL, tailoring the treatment, and understanding the potential prognosis for each patient.

DESCRIBE A TYPICAL WORKUP FOR ALL

The initial evaluation for ALL begins with a thorough medical history and physical examination. This helps doctors understand the patient's symptoms and overall health. Laboratory tests are essential, including a complete blood count (CBC) to check for abnormal blood cells, a blood chemistry profile to assess organ function, liver function tests, and a coagulation panel to evaluate blood clotting. Additionally, a tumor lysis syndrome (TLS) panel is done to monitor harmful substances released when leukemia cells break down. Pregnancy tests are performed for females of childbearing potential, and for males, a testicular ultrasound may be conducted to check for leukemia involvement in the testes, although this is rare.

Fertility considerations are also important, as treatments like chemotherapy can affect reproductive health. Doctors offer counseling on fertility preservation options, such as sperm or egg freezing, before treatment begins. Imaging studies, including CT or MRI of the head, chest X-rays, and whole-body PET/CT scans, are performed to check for spread of leukemia to the brain, chest, or other parts of the body. A lumbar puncture is done to evaluate if leukemia has affected the spinal fluid. Cardiac health is assessed through an echocardiogram, as chemotherapy can impact heart function, especially in patients with a history of heart problems.

Genetic testing is sometimes necessary to identify any hereditary factors that might affect treatment decisions. In cases of high-risk ALL, such as those with low chromosome counts, testing for specific genetic mutations like TP53 may be recommended. Additionally, a family history of cancer can help doctors assess the risk of inherited cancer syndromes. Infection checks are crucial, as patients with ALL may have a weakened immune system. This comprehensive workup helps doctors determine the best treatment plan, monitor the disease's progression, and address any other health issues the patient may face.

GENETIC ABNORMALITIES AND MOLECULAR SUBTYPES OF ALL

Certain genetic changes in the leukemia cells play an important role in understanding the disease, determining the patient's risk, and planning the best treatment. For B-cell ALL (B-ALL), some common genetic changes include:

- Hyperdiploidy: Having extra chromosomes (51–67 chromosomes).
- Hypodiploidy: Having fewer chromosomes (<44 chromosomes).
- BCR::ABL1 fusion (also known as the Philadelphia chromosome)
- KMT2A rearrangement
- ETV6::RUNX1 fusion
- TCF3::PBX1 fusion

There are also other specific genetic changes that can affect how the leukemia behaves and how it should be treated, such as rearrangements of DUX4, MEF2D, and ZNF384, or changes in genes like MYC and PAX5.

In cases where the leukemia doesn't respond well to treatment, especially when the MYC gene is involved, doctors might consider treating the patient like they have a different type of cancer called mature B-cell lymphoma.

The World Health Organization (WHO) updated the classification of ALL in 2016, adding new subtypes, including:

- BCR::ABL1-like ALL: A subtype of B-ALL that has certain genetic features similar to another type of leukemia.
- iAMP21: A rare subtype of B-ALL with an extra copy of chromosome 21.
- ETP lymphoblastic leukemia: A specific form of T-ALL with unique genetic features.
- Natural killer (NK) cell leukemia/lymphoma: A rare form of leukemia involving NK cells.

Doctors use genetic tests to identify these abnormalities and help predict the likely outcome of the disease and which treatments will work best. Some genetic changes are linked to a better response to treatment, while others are associated with more challenging outcomes. These findings help guide treatment decisions for each patient.

Favorable-Risk Features

For children with ALL, certain genetic changes are linked to a better chance of recovery. One of the most common changes in childhood ALL is hyperdiploidy, which means the leukemia cells have more than the usual number of chromosomes (51 to 67 chromosomes). This happens in about 25% of childhood B-cell ALL cases, but it's much rarer in adults (only about 7%). Another helpful genetic change in children is ETV6::RUNX1, a specific gene rearrangement that happens in 25% of cases of childhood ALL, but only about 2% of adults with ALL. These genetic changes are usually associated with better treatment outcomes in children, and are seen less often in adolescents and young adults compared to younger children.

Intermediate-Risk Features

There are other genetic changes that are less clear but may indicate an intermediate risk. These include changes like MEF2D rearrangement, ZNF384 rearrangement, and PAX5 mutations. These abnormalities are still being studied to understand how they affect the outcome of ALL and whether they represent a higher or lower risk for patients. More research is needed to fully understand the significance of these genetic features.

Unfavorable-Risk Features

Some genetic changes in ALL are linked to a higher risk of poor outcomes. These include:

1. Hypodiploidy: This means having fewer chromosomes than normal. It can be further divided into different categories based on how many chromosomes are missing. It occurs in about 1-2% of children with ALL and is often associated with a poor prognosis. This condition can sometimes be difficult to distinguish from another type of

genetic change, so more tests are needed for accurate diagnosis.

2. KMT2A Rearrangements: This genetic change, often found in infants, happens in around 5% of childhood ALL cases. It is linked to poor outcomes, especially in very young children.

3. T-cell Fusion Genes (TCF3::HLF, TCF4::HLF): These rare genetic changes (less than 1% of ALL cases) are linked to poor outcomes. Some specific gene fusions, like TCF3::PBX1, are associated with intermediate outcomes.

4. iAMP21: This involves the amplification of a part of chromosome 21. It occurs in about 2% of childhood ALL cases and is associated with a poor prognosis if treated with less aggressive treatment.

5. BCR::ABL1: This genetic change is found in about 2% of childhood ALL cases but is more common in adults (about 25%). It is linked to a poor prognosis, although younger children with this change tend to do better than adolescents.

6. IKZF1 Mutations: Mutations in the IKZF1 gene are seen in about 15-20% of pediatric B-ALL cases and are often associated with a higher chance of relapse.

7. BCR::ABL1-like ALL: This subtype occurs in about 15% of pediatric B-ALL cases and has a poor prognosis. It shares similar genetic features with BCR::ABL1-positive ALL but

lacks the BCR::ABL1 fusion gene. Patients with this subtype may benefit from targeted therapies, such as tyrosine kinase inhibitors (TKIs), which are designed to block the abnormal signaling pathways caused by these genetic changes.

Genetic abnormalities in T-ALL

T-ALL (T-cell acute lymphoblastic leukemia) is often linked to certain genetic changes that affect how cells grow and divide. One of the main changes is mutations in the NOTCH1 gene, which are found in more than half of T-ALL cases. These mutations help the cancer cells grow and avoid normal controls that would stop them. Additionally, some cases of T-ALL have mutations in FBXW7, a gene that affects NOTCH1, leading to even more uncontrolled cell growth. Around 10-15% of T-ALL cases have this change.

Interestingly, these mutations in NOTCH1 and FBXW7 are usually associated with a better outcome and lower levels of minimal residual disease (MRD), which means fewer cancer cells are left after treatment. However, it's still unclear if these mutations alone can predict how well a patient will do or if other factors, like mutations in RAS or PTEN, need to be considered as well.

By studying these genetic and molecular changes,

doctors can better understand the type of T-ALL and how likely it is to respond to treatment.

Tests used to identify genetic abnormalities

To help doctors understand the genetic makeup of leukemia, several methods are used to identify recurring genetic changes. These include:

1. Karyotyping: A test that directly looks at the chromosomes in cells to find any abnormal changes.
2. FISH (Fluorescence in Situ Hybridization): This test checks for specific genetic abnormalities by using special probes that light up when they find targeted genetic changes.
3. RT-PCR (Reverse Transcriptase-Polymerase Chain Reaction): This method helps detect gene fusions, like the BCR::ABL1 fusion in B-ALL, which has different versions (such as p190 and p210).
4. Next-Generation Sequencing (NGS): A more advanced method that looks at many genes at once to find changes in DNA.

Doctors may also test for additional gene fusions and mutations, especially for BCR::ABL1-like ALL. These include mutations in genes like ABL1, CRLF2, JAK2, and others that can help determine the best treatment approach.

To identify hidden genetic changes, doctors may use special probes or NGS-based tests. In some cases, microarrays or whole transcriptome sequencing are used to detect rare subtypes of leukemia based on their gene expression patterns.

PROGNOSTIC FACTORS AND RISK STRATIFICATION

Unlike solid tumors, Acute Lymphoblastic Leukemia (ALL) does not have traditional "stages" like cancers of the breast, lung, or colon. Instead, ALL is classified based on **risk factors, genetic features, and response to therapy**. These classifications guide treatment but are not referred to as stages. Doctors use a risk assessment system to decide how intense a child's treatment for acute lymphoblastic leukemia needs to be. Different groups of experts—like the Children's Oncology Group (COG) in the U.S., St. Jude Children's Research Hospital, and the Dana-Farber Cancer Institute—have worked together to classify ALL into low-risk, standard-risk, high-risk, or very-high-risk categories.

What Determines Risk?

Doctors consider several factors about the patient and the leukemia:

1. Age – Children between 1 and 10 years old tend to have a better prognosis.
2. White Blood Cell Count (WBC) – A WBC count below 50,000 is considered standard risk.
3. Type of Leukemia Cells (B-ALL or T-ALL) –

   - B-ALL is classified based on genetic findings. Certain changes in the leukemia cells make it high-risk, like:

- A specific gene change called BCR-ABL1 (also known as the Philadelphia chromosome).
- Hypodiploidy, meaning fewer than 44 chromosomes.
- KMT2A gene rearrangements, often seen in babies under 1 year.
- Poor response to the first round of treatment.
- Other findings, like extra chromosomes (hyperdiploidy) or a gene change called ETV6::RUNX1, mean a better chance of cure (lower risk).

4. Response to Treatment –
- Doctors measure how quickly the leukemia goes away.
- They use a test called minimal residual disease (MRD) to see if cancer cells remain after treatment. Low MRD means a better response.

How Risk Groups Affect Treatment

- Low or Standard Risk: These patients typically have less intense treatment.
- High or Very-High Risk: More intense treatment is used to ensure the leukemia doesn't come back.

Who Decides the Risk?

Groups like the Children's Oncology Group (COG), St. Jude, and Dana-Farber use similar systems to assess risk. In Europe, the Berlin-Frankfurt-Münster (BFM) Group also looks at how the leukemia responds to certain drugs (like prednisone) and genetic findings to decide risk.

Doctors may reassess risk after the first phase of treatment (induction therapy) to make sure the child is getting the right therapy.

Let's explore the topic of prognostication in greater detail. There are numerous approaches to this subject, each offering unique insights. Below, we discuss the salient points of the most significant and widely recognized methods.

1. Children's Oncology Group (COG) Approach:
In the COG approach, children with B-cell ALL are initially classified into two groups: standard-risk or high-risk. A child is considered standard risk if they are between 1 and 10 years old and their white blood cell (WBC) count is less than 50,000. If a child is 10 years or older or has a WBC count above 50,000, they fall into the high-risk group. Other high-risk factors include cancer in the brain or spinal fluid (CNS-3), testicular disease, the presence of a gene change called BCR-ABL1 (Philadelphia chromosome), or receiving steroids before starting treatment.

After the first phase of treatment (induction), doctors use a test called minimal residual disease (MRD) to see how much leukemia remains. MRD helps further refine risk into favorable, average, or high risk. The lower the MRD, the better the response. For example, MRD below 0.01% is now considered a good result. Children with T-cell ALL (T-ALL) are assessed primarily based on whether leukemia has spread outside the bone marrow (extramedullary disease) and their MRD levels after treatment. For T-ALL, MRD at the end of induction (day 29) and during consolidation is key; if MRD is above 0.1%, the risk increases.

2. St. Jude Consortium Approach:

The St. Jude approach initially classifies children with ALL into low-risk or standard-risk groups. A child is considered low risk if they have B-ALL with good features, such as a DNA index of 1.16 or higher or a specific gene change called ETV6::RUNX1. Children aged 1 to 9.9 years with a WBC count below 50,000 also fall into this group.

Children are considered standard risk if they are 10 years or older, have a WBC count above 50,000, or show other high-risk features like leukemia spreading to the brain (CNS-3), testicles, or adverse genetic changes (e.g., BCR-ABL1, KMT2A rearrangement, or iAMP21). T-ALL is automatically placed in the standard-risk category. After induction treatment, MRD becomes critical again: children with ≥1% MRD by day 15 or ≥0.01% MRD at the end of induction are monitored closely. If MRD remains high or increases during treatment, the disease is reclassified as high risk.

3. Dana-Farber Cancer Institute (DFCI) Approach:

In the DFCI approach, children are first assigned to risk groups early—by day 10 of treatment—using tests like FISH, karyotyping, and advanced genetic

panels. Children are placed into three groups:
- Standard risk: Ages 1 to 15, WBC count less than 50,000, and no high-risk genetic features.
- High risk: Includes children with the BCR-ABL1 gene, a condition called iAMP21, or T-ALL.
- Very high risk: Includes children with aggressive genetic features such as IKZF1 deletion, KMT2A rearrangement, low hypodiploidy (fewer than normal chromosomes), or the gene change TCF3::HLF.

After induction treatment, MRD levels help refine risk. Children with low MRD (below 0.01%) are considered low or standard risk. High MRD or persistent leukemia after treatment indicates high or very high risk.

WHAT ARE THE KEY TREATMENT PHASES AND THERAPEUTIC AGENTS TO CONSIDER IN MANAGING ALL?

The treatment for acute lymphoblastic leukemia is one of the most intensive in cancer care, but it has been carefully developed to maximize the chances of cure. While the exact details—like the choice of drugs and treatment duration—can vary depending on age, risk level, and leukemia subtype, the general treatment plan is divided into three main phases:

1. Induction
2. Consolidation
3. Maintenance

Some treatment plans have additional detailed phases like intensification or involve targeted therapy and, in some cases, a stem cell transplant (HCT). Throughout treatment, protection of the central nervous system (CNS) is a critical part of the plan to prevent leukemia from spreading to the brain or spinal fluid.

Phases in ALL treatment are essential to effectively target the disease at different stages, ensuring optimal outcomes. Each phase—induction, consolidation, and maintenance—serves a specific purpose: induction aims to achieve remission by eliminating most leukemic cells, consolidation reduces the risk of relapse by targeting any remaining disease, and maintenance prevents recurrence by suppressing residual leukemia over time. This stepwise approach maximizes the chances of cure while minimizing treatment-related toxicity.

The duration of each phase in ALL treatment can vary based on patient age, risk stratification, and treatment protocols, but typically follows this timeline:

1. Induction Phase: Usually lasts 4 to 6 weeks. The goal is to achieve complete remission by eliminating most leukemic cells.
2. Consolidation Phase: This phase often spans 4 to 6 months, focusing on eradicating residual disease and preventing relapse. This phase may include an intensification phase in some protocols.
3. Maintenance Phase: Generally continues for 2 to 3 years in most pediatric cases and slightly shorter for adults. It involves lower-intensity therapy to sustain remission and prevent recurrence.

These durations can vary depending on specific treatment regimens and patient responses.

Induction Phase

The induction phase is the first and most critical step of treatment. The goal is to reduce the leukemia cells in the bone marrow as much as possible and achieve remission. Induction chemotherapy typically includes several drugs:

- Vincristine
- Corticosteroids like prednisone or dexamethasone
- Asparaginase
- Sometimes anthracyclines like daunorubicin (for higher-risk patients).

For standard-risk children, induction may involve three drugs, while higher-risk patients often receive a more intensive four-drug combination. In some adult and older adolescent (AYA) patients, an even more intensive five-drug regimen may be used.

Research has shown that dexamethasone is better than prednisone for reducing the risk of leukemia spreading to the brain (CNS relapse) and improving long-term outcomes. However, dexamethasone can also cause side effects like bone damage (osteonecrosis) and increased risk of infection. Doctors carefully weigh the risks and benefits when choosing corticosteroids.

For asparaginase, several forms are available, including:
- Pegaspargase, which has a long half-life but is now limited to certain age groups.
- Calaspargase, preferred for most children because it lasts longer in the body.
- Erwinia asparaginase, used when patients have an allergic reaction to other forms.

Consolidation Phase

After remission is achieved during induction,

the consolidation phase aims to eliminate any remaining leukemia cells that may still be in the body. This phase is more intensive for high-risk patients and can last up to 8 months. Drugs used in this phase include:
- Methotrexate (often given at high doses)
- Cytarabine
- 6-mercaptopurine (6-MP)
- Vincristine
- Corticosteroids
- Asparaginase

Some treatment plans also include drugs like 6-thioguanine (6-TG), particularly in later phases called delayed intensification.

Maintenance Phase

The goal of the maintenance phase is to keep the leukemia from coming back (relapse) after induction and consolidation. This phase is usually less intensive and lasts about 2 to 3 years. The most common drugs used include:
- 6-Mercaptopurine (6-MP) taken daily.
- Methotrexate given weekly.
- Periodic doses of vincristine and corticosteroids.

Special Considerations for 6-MP
- Some patients may process 6-MP differently due to their genetics. Doctors often check for changes in genes like TPMT and NUDT15 to adjust dosing and avoid serious side effects like low blood counts.
- For some patients, especially teenagers and young

adults, nonadherence (not taking the medication as prescribed) can be an issue. If blood counts don't drop despite increasing doses, doctors may suspect nonadherence and work with families to address it.

Monitoring and Adherence

Throughout all treatment phases, careful monitoring is essential. Doctors check the minimal residual disease (MRD) to see how well treatment is working and make adjustments if needed. Adherence to medication is especially important during maintenance therapy to prevent relapse. If needed, doctors may measure drug levels in the blood or perform pill counts to ensure patients are receiving the right amount of medication.

HOW CAN EXTRAMEDULLARY DISEASE BE PREVENTED AND TREATED IN ALL?

Extramedullary disease means leukemia cells are found outside the bone marrow, like in the brain and spinal fluid (CNS) or the testes. Because regular chemotherapy cannot easily reach these areas due to natural barriers like the blood-brain barrier and blood-testis barrier, doctors use specific therapies to target these areas and prevent relapse.

For the CNS, treatment includes:
- Intrathecal (IT) therapy: Chemotherapy (like methotrexate, cytarabine, or corticosteroids) is injected directly into the spinal fluid.
- Cranial radiation: In some cases, radiation is used to target leukemia cells in the brain.
- Systemic chemotherapy: High-dose treatments like methotrexate, cytarabine, and asparaginase help clear leukemia cells throughout the body, including the CNS.

CNS treatment and prevention occur throughout all phases of ALL treatment—induction, consolidation, and maintenance—to keep the disease from returning. For children with leukemia in the testes at diagnosis that doesn't improve after the first phase of treatment, doctors may use radiation therapy to treat the testes.

WHAT IS THE ROLE OF HEMATOPOIETIC CELL TRANSPLANTATION (HCT) IN THE TREATMENT OF ALL?

Stem cell transplantation (HCT) is an option for children with high-risk ALL or leukemia that doesn't respond well to treatment. It involves replacing diseased bone marrow with healthy stem cells from a donor. Donors can be:
- Matched family members
- Unrelated donors
- Umbilical cord blood donors
- Partially matched (haploidentical) donors.

Both total body irradiation (TBI) (radiation to the whole body) and non-TBI chemotherapy regimens are used to prepare for the transplant. Research shows TBI works better for many children, but non-TBI options are still being studied. For infants, the decision to use HCT is complex but may be considered in high-risk cases, especially when leukemia has certain gene changes like KMT2A rearrangements.

HCT is a potentially life-saving treatment for ALL, particularly in high-risk or relapsed cases. However, its safety depends on several factors, including the patient's overall health, age, disease status, and the type of transplant. While HCT carries risks such as graft-versus-host disease (GVHD), infections, and organ toxicity, advances in supportive care and conditioning regimens have significantly improved its safety and outcomes. Careful patient selection and monitoring are key to minimizing risks and optimizing benefits.

WHAT IS THE ROLE OF TARGETED THERAPIES IN THE TREATMENT OF ALL?

New targeted therapies have transformed the treatment of ALL, especially for patients with high-risk genetic changes or relapsed/refractory disease (leukemia that returns or doesn't respond to treatment).

Key examples include:
1. Tyrosine Kinase Inhibitors (TKIs): These are used for BCR-ABL1-positive ALL (Philadelphia chromosome-positive leukemia). TKIs (like imatinib and dasatinib) block signals that help leukemia cells grow.
   - Important note: Some stomach medications (like PPIs) can interfere with TKI absorption, so doctors carefully manage these combinations.

2. Janus Kinase (JAK) Inhibitors: These are being tested for BCR-ABL1-like ALL cases with specific genetic changes, like CRLF2 and JAK mutations.

3. Nelarabine: Approved for treating T-ALL that has relapsed or is hard to treat.

4. Monoclonal Antibodies: These therapies target proteins on leukemia cells:
   - Examples include rituximab (CD20), inotuzumab ozogamicin (CD22), and blinatumomab (a bispecific antibody that targets CD19).

5. CAR T-Cell Therapy: This is a breakthrough treatment where a patient's immune cells (T cells) are engineered to attack leukemia cells. CAR T cells targeting CD19 have shown promising results, especially for children and young adults with relapsed or hard-to-treat B-ALL.

Targeted therapies can be used during induction, consolidation, maintenance, or when the leukemia relapses. They offer more precise treatment options and are improving survival outcomes for many patients.

WHAT ARE THE KEY TREATMENT CONSIDERATIONS FOR ADOLESCENT AND YOUNG ADULT (AYA) PATIENTS WITH ALL?

Adolescents and young adults (AYA) with ALL, typically aged 15–21 years, can be treated with either pediatric or adult protocols, depending on the institution. Studies have shown that AYA patients treated on pediatric protocols have much better outcomes, with higher survival rates, compared to those treated on adult regimens. This is because pediatric protocols use higher doses of chemotherapy and more intense treatment targeting the central nervous system (CNS).

However, AYA patients still have poorer outcomes compared to younger children under age 10. This is due to both biological and social factors:
- AYA patients have fewer favorable genetic features, such as hyperdiploidy or the ETV6::RUNX1 mutation, which are common in younger children.
- They also have a higher chance of having poor-risk genetic changes, like the BCR-ABL1 gene (Philadelphia chromosome), hypodiploidy, or early T-cell precursor ALL (ETP-ALL).
- Chemotherapy resistance: Leukemia cells in AYA patients are more resistant to chemotherapy compared to those in younger children. This often results in a slower response to treatment.

Additionally, social challenges impact AYA outcomes. Fewer AYA patients enroll in clinical trials compared to younger children (only 2% vs. 60%), and they may face issues like lower treatment adherence and limited access to health insurance. Younger children often benefit from parental supervision, which helps ensure better compliance with treatment schedules.

WHAT ARE THE TREATMENT CHALLENGES AND CONSIDERATIONS FOR VULNERABLE POPULATIONS IN ALL?

Infants and children with Down syndrome are considered vulnerable populations in the treatment of pediatric ALL due to their unique clinical challenges and increased treatment sensitivity.

Infants (<12 months old)

Infants with ALL represent a high-risk group because their leukemia often doesn't respond well to treatment, and they face more treatment-related complications. They are also at a higher risk for early relapse in the bone marrow, CNS, and other areas. Some common challenges in infants include:
- High white blood cell (WBC) counts at diagnosis
- Massive organ enlargement (organomegaly)
- Low platelet counts (thrombocytopenia)
- CNS leukemia at diagnosis
- A genetic change called KMT2A rearrangement (the most common genetic abnormality in infant ALL).

Due to these risks, infants require very carefully designed treatment plans to balance intense therapy with the need to manage complications.

Children with Down syndrome (trisomy 21)

Children with Down syndrome have a higher risk

of developing ALL, although the exact reason is unknown. Their leukemia often has unique characteristics:
- It rarely occurs in infants under 1 year of age.
- They have a lower incidence of both favorable and unfavorable genetic changes compared to children without Down syndrome.
- They are more sensitive to methotrexate (MTX) and more susceptible to infections during treatment.

Children with Down syndrome may also have leukemia that expresses CRLF2, a gene linked to JAK2 mutations, which can affect treatment response. Historically, outcomes for children with Down syndrome and ALL were worse due to treatment complications and challenges following protocols. However, recent data suggest that if the treatment is carefully tailored and includes strong supportive care (like infection management), these children can achieve outcomes similar to other patients with ALL.

HOW IS MINIMAL RESIDUAL DISEASE (MRD) USED TO GUIDE TREATMENT DECISIONS IN ALL?

Minimal Residual Disease (MRD) refers to small numbers of leukemia cells that remain in the body after treatment but are too few to detect using standard tests. These cells are often the cause of relapse (when the disease comes back).

Doctors use special tests to measure MRD with high accuracy. These include:
1. Flow Cytometry: Detects leukemia-specific markers on cells.
2. PCR (Polymerase Chain Reaction): Identifies tiny amounts of leukemia-related genes, like BCR-ABL1 or clonal rearrangements in the immune system's Ig/TCR genes.
3. Next-Generation Sequencing (NGS): A newer, highly sensitive method that can detect MRD levels as low as 0.0001% (1 in 1 million cells).

Studies have shown that MRD is a strong predictor of outcomes in children and adults with ALL. If MRD levels remain high after treatment, there is a greater risk of relapse. On the other hand, patients who clear MRD quickly have much better long-term outcomes.

For example:
- End of Induction (EOI) MRD is often checked to

assess how well the first phase of treatment is working.
- Low MRD (<0.01%) at the EOI is a good sign and is linked to higher survival rates.
- High MRD (>0.01%) may require stronger or different treatment to prevent relapse.

MRD is typically measured at specific times during treatment:
1. End of Induction Therapy (around day 29): To evaluate the response to initial chemotherapy.
2. End of Consolidation Therapy: To check for any remaining disease.
3. Before a Stem Cell Transplant (HCT): MRD levels help decide if further treatment is needed before the transplant.
4. During Maintenance Therapy or Follow-up: In some cases, MRD is monitored to look for early signs of relapse.

MRD in Different Patient Groups

- Children with B-ALL: Studies show that patients with MRD positivity (>0.01%) at the end of induction or later have a much higher risk of relapse compared to MRD-negative patients.
- T-ALL: MRD is also very important for children with T-ALL. High MRD levels (e.g., >0.1%) at specific time points are associated with poorer outcomes.
- Infants with KMT2A Rearrangements: Infants often have high-risk disease, and MRD levels at the end of induction and end of consolidation strongly

predict survival outcomes.

How MRD Affects Treatment Decisions

Doctors use MRD results to adjust treatment based on a patient's risk of relapse:

1. MRD-Negative Patients: Patients with very low or undetectable MRD may be able to receive less intensive therapy to reduce side effects.
2. MRD-Positive Patients: High MRD levels may indicate the need for:
   - Stronger chemotherapy.
   - Stem cell transplantation (HCT) to reduce relapse risk.
   - Targeted therapies (e.g., CAR T-cell therapy or monoclonal antibodies) to eliminate MRD.

In some studies, MRD-guided treatment has improved survival, especially in patients with a higher risk of relapse.

How is MRD Tested?

- Bone Marrow Samples: The most accurate MRD measurements come from bone marrow, usually collected at key time points in treatment.
- Blood Samples: In some cases, MRD can be checked in the blood, but bone marrow remains the gold standard for testing.
- Advanced Testing (NGS): Newer methods like NGS-based MRD testing are very sensitive and are particularly helpful after therapies like CAR T-cell therapy.

By carefully monitoring MRD throughout treatment, doctors can provide a personalized treatment plan that improves the chances of long-term survival while minimizing unnecessary side effects.

HOW IS BCR::ABL1-NEGATIVE OR BCR::ABL1-LIKE B-ALL MANAGED?

The principles of managing all types of ALL follow a structured, stepwise approach that remains consistent across subtypes. Treatment is divided into **three main phases**: induction, consolidation (may include intensification), and maintenance. Each phase is designed to achieve specific goals —induction aims to achieve complete remission, consolidation seeks to eliminate residual disease and prevent relapse, and maintenance provides long-term suppression of any remaining leukemia cells to sustain remission.

At **predefined time points** during treatment, careful **evaluation of disease response** is performed. This includes assessments such as bone marrow examinations, minimal residual disease (MRD) monitoring, and clinical response evaluations. These results are critical as they guide further therapy decisions. If a patient shows suboptimal response or evidence of persistent disease, the treatment plan may be **modified or intensified**. This could include changing chemotherapy agents, incorporating targeted therapies, or considering hematopoietic cell transplantation (HCT) for high-risk or refractory cases.

Depending on the specific type of ALL,

modifications are made in treatment planning to address the unique biological and clinical features of each subtype. ALL is a heterogeneous disease, with variations such as B-cell ALL, T-cell ALL, and specific genetic subtypes like BCR::ABL1-positive or BCR::ABL1-like ALL.

BCR::ABL1-negative B-ALL refers to a form of acute lymphoblastic leukemia that **does not carry the Philadelphia chromosome** (BCR::ABL1 fusion). A subset called BCR::ABL1-like B-ALL has similar gene expression patterns but without the BCR::ABL1 fusion and is associated with higher risk and poor outcomes.

The treatment of this leukemia has been improved through large clinical trials in children, adolescents, and young adults (AYA). Below are simplified highlights of major trials that guide current treatment strategies.

Children's Oncology Group (COG) Trials

1. COG AALL0331 and AALL0932
- Goal: Optimize treatment for standard-risk B-ALL.
- Patients were treated with a 3-drug induction (dexamethasone, vincristine, pegaspargase) and grouped into risk categories based on genetic markers and early response to treatment.
- Key Findings:
  - Patients with MRD >0.01% at the end of induction (EOI) benefited from intensified therapy.
  - Higher methotrexate doses and less frequent

steroid pulses during maintenance did not improve outcomes.
- Survival Rates: 6-year survival was excellent at 96%.

2. COG AALL0232 and AALL1131
- These trials focused on high-risk B-ALL.
- Key Findings:
  - High-dose methotrexate (HD-MTX) improved survival compared to standard methotrexate.
  - Dexamethasone was better for children <10 years but caused more bone complications in older patients.
  - Triple intrathecal (IT) therapy did not improve CNS outcomes over standard IT methotrexate.
  - New agents like dasatinib (for ABL-class lesions) and ruxolitinib (for JAK-STAT mutations) are being studied.

Dana-Farber Cancer Institute (DFCI) ALL Protocols

1. DFCI 05-001
- Introduced a risk classification system using MRD levels and adverse genetics.
- Patients with high MRD or poor genetic features (e.g., KMT2A rearrangement) were treated with more intensive therapy.
- Key Findings:
  - 5-year survival rates were 87% overall, with lower survival in very-high-risk groups.
  - Patients aged 15 years or older had worse outcomes, highlighting the need for targeted

strategies.

2. DFCI 11-001
- Compared two forms of asparaginase: calaspargase and pegaspargase. Both were equally effective, with similar safety profiles.

3. Ongoing DFCI Trials
- Current studies focus on better risk classification using NGS-based MRD testing and new markers like IKZF1 deletion.

St. Jude Total Therapy Studies

1. Total XV Study
- Key Aim: To safely omit cranial radiation as CNS prophylaxis.
- Patients were treated with multi-drug chemotherapy and risk-stratified using MRD.
- Key Findings:
  - Cranial radiation was safely avoided without compromising survival.
  - 5-year survival rates were excellent (93.5%).

2. Total XVI Study
- Investigated the impact of higher doses of pegaspargase and early CNS-directed therapy for patients at high risk of CNS relapse.
- Key Findings:
  - Higher doses of pegaspargase did not improve outcomes.
  - Early CNS treatment significantly reduced CNS relapses.

3. Ongoing Total XVII Study
- Focuses on precision medicine based on genomic findings. New treatments being studied include:
    - Dasatinib for patients with ABL-class fusions.
    - Ruxolitinib for patients with JAK-STAT pathway mutations.

Role of Blinatumomab

Blinatumomab is a bispecific T-cell engager (BiTE) antibody that helps the body's immune system fight leukemia. It works by:
- Binding to CD19 on leukemia cells.
- Simultaneously activating CD3-positive T cells, which then target and destroy the leukemia cells.

Blinatumomab is particularly useful for patients with minimal residual disease (MRD) after chemotherapy or those with relapsed/refractory B-ALL.

Studies have shown that blinatumomab is highly effective in patients with persistent MRD (leukemia cells remaining at very low levels after chemotherapy).

1. Key Results:
   - In patients with MRD ≥0.01%, blinatumomab cleared MRD in up to 88% of cases after one cycle.
   - Many patients who achieved MRD negativity went on to receive a stem cell transplant (HCT), further improving their chances of long-term remission.

2. FDA Approval:
- Blinatumomab is approved for patients (adults and children) with MRD ≥0.1% who are in their first or second remission (CR1 or CR2).

Newer studies are exploring how blinatumomab can be used earlier in treatment to improve outcomes.

1. ECOG-ACRIN E1910 Trial (Phase III)
- This trial tested whether blinatumomab could improve survival in adults (ages 30–70) with newly diagnosed BCR::ABL1-negative B-ALL.
- Patients who achieved MRD negativity after induction chemotherapy were randomized to receive either:
    - Standard chemotherapy alone, or
    - Blinatumomab plus chemotherapy.
- Results:
    - The addition of blinatumomab significantly improved survival rates:
        - 3-Year Overall Survival (OS): 85% (blinatumomab) vs. 68% (chemotherapy alone).
        - 3-Year Relapse-Free Survival (RFS): 80% (blinatumomab) vs. 64% (chemotherapy alone).
    - Conclusion: Blinatumomab significantly improves outcomes, even in patients who are MRD-negative.

Ongoing trials are investigating blinatumomab in combination with chemotherapy to see if it further reduces relapse risk, particularly in high-risk B-ALL.

HCT

For children and young adults with high-risk B-ALL, allogeneic stem cell transplant may be considered if:
1. MRD remains positive at the end of consolidation (EOC).
2. High-risk genetic features (e.g., hypodiploidy) are present alongside MRD positivity at the end of induction (EOI).

Stem cell transplant provides an option for long-term remission in these high-risk cases, though it is often recommended in the context of a clinical trial for certain subtypes like hypodiploid B-ALL.

Guidelines

The most widely accepted guidelines recommend that pediatric and adolescent/young adult (AYA) patients with BCR::ABL1-negative or BCR::ABL1-like ALL be treated in a clinical trial whenever possible. Clinical trials often offer the most advanced treatments and help improve outcomes.

If a clinical trial isn't available, treatment follows these steps:

1. Induction Therapy:
   - Patients are treated with multi-drug chemotherapy to achieve remission.
   - If MRD (Minimal Residual Disease) testing shows no remaining leukemia cells (MRD-negative

CR), treatment continues with risk-based therapy tailored to the patient's risk level.

2. Post-Induction Treatment: If MRD is negative at the end of induction, the appropriate consolidation phase, followed by the maintenance phase, is initiated based on the patient's initial risk group.

Note that:
- Patients with MRD-positive CR (leukemia cells remain at a low level):
  - May receive intensified consolidation therapy (stronger treatment).
  - Blinatumomab (an immunotherapy drug) can also be added to help clear the remaining leukemia.
- If MRD remains positive after consolidation, options include:
- Blinatumomab again.
- Tisagenlecleucel (CAR T-cell therapy), preferably as part of a clinical trial.

3. Stem Cell Transplant (HCT):
  - HCT may be considered during consolidation or maintenance therapy, especially for high-risk patients.
  - After CAR T-cell therapy (like tisagenlecleucel), many patients remain in remission without HCT, as the CAR T cells can keep leukemia under control.

4. Refractory Disease:

- If a patient does not achieve remission (less than CR) after induction, the disease is treated as refractory with more advanced therapies.

How is relapsed or refractory BCR::ABL1-negative or BCR::ABL1-like ALL managed?

What is Relapsed or Refractory ALL?

- Relapsed ALL: The leukemia comes back after treatment.
- Refractory ALL: The leukemia does not respond well to initial treatment.

For pediatric patients, outcomes for R/R ALL have historically been poor. Success depends on factors like how soon the relapse happens and whether the patient achieved a long remission after their first treatment (CR1).

General Principles for Treating R/R B-ALL

1. Early Relapse (<36 months): These cases are harder to treat and usually require stem cell transplant (HCT) for a chance at cure.
2. Late Relapse (≥36 months): Chemotherapy alone may be enough, though HCT may still be considered.

New therapies, including immunotherapy (like Blinatumomab and CAR T cells) and targeted agents (like Inotuzumab Ozogamicin), are now helping improve outcomes.

Key Treatment Strategies for R/R B-ALL

1. Chemotherapy-Based Regimens

- ALL-REZ BFM 90 Trial:
  - Multi-drug chemotherapy achieved remission in 83–100% of patients, especially those with late relapses.
  - HCT further improved outcomes for those in second remission (CR2).

- COG AALL01P2 Study:
  - Patients received three blocks of chemotherapy.
  - MRD negativity (no detectable disease) after the first month of treatment predicted better outcomes.

- Clofarabine and Fludarabine Regimens:
  - Drugs like clofarabine and fludarabine are often combined with other chemotherapy agents to treat R/R ALL.
  - These regimens can achieve remission in up to 76% of patients.

2. Immunotherapy

Blinatumomab
- How it works: It connects immune T cells to leukemia cells to destroy them.
- Studies show:
  - Blinatumomab achieved MRD negativity in many patients and helped prepare them for stem cell transplant.
  - In pediatric patients, Blinatumomab improved survival and allowed more patients to proceed to

HCT compared to standard chemotherapy.

CAR T-Cell Therapy (e.g., Tisagenlecleucel)
- What it is: A patient's own T cells are genetically engineered to recognize and kill leukemia cells carrying the CD19 protein.
- Results:
  - High remission rates (81–90%) in children and young adults.
  - Some patients stay in long-term remission without needing a transplant.
- Side Effects:
  - Cytokine Release Syndrome (CRS): A severe immune reaction that can cause fever, low blood pressure, and breathing issues.
  - Neurotoxicity: Temporary confusion, seizures, or speech problems.
  - These side effects are treatable with medications like tocilizumab and steroids.

Inotuzumab Ozogamicin (InO)
- What it is: A targeted drug that delivers chemotherapy directly to leukemia cells carrying the CD22 protein.
- Key Findings:
  - InO achieved remission in about 80% of patients with relapsed B-ALL.
  - Risk: InO can cause sinusoidal obstruction syndrome (SOS), a serious liver condition, especially in patients receiving HCT.
  - Prevention: Doctors may use a medication like ursodiol to help protect the liver.

3. Stem Cell Transplant (HCT)
For patients with early relapse or those who remain MRD-positive, HCT remains the most established curative option.
- HCT involves replacing diseased bone marrow with healthy stem cells from a donor.
- While HCT has risks (e.g., infections, graft-versus-host disease), it offers a chance for long-term remission.

Guidelines

For patients whose leukemia comes back (relapse) or does not respond to treatment:

1. First Relapse:
   - Initial treatment includes systemic chemotherapy to get the disease into remission.
   - If a patient achieves remission (CR2):
     - MRD Negative: Options include:
       - Blinatumomab or continued chemotherapy.
     - Maintenance therapy or stem cell transplant (HCT) to lower the chance of relapse.
     - MRD Positive: Options include:
       - Blinatumomab, tisagenlecleucel (CAR T-cell therapy), or Inotuzumab ozogamicin (InO) before proceeding to HCT.

2. Multiple Relapses or Less Than CR:
   - Treatment options include:
     - Chemotherapy.

- Immunotherapies like Blinatumomab, Tisagenlecleucel, or Inotuzumab Ozogamicin (InO).

- Mini-hyper-CVD (a less intense chemotherapy regimen).

- If the leukemia responds to treatment, a stem cell transplant (HCT) may follow to provide a chance for long-term remission.

3. CAR T-Cell Therapy:

- Tisagenlecleucel can help some patients achieve long-term remission without needing a stem cell transplant. However, the role of HCT after CAR T-cell therapy remains unclear.

4. When the Disease Does Not Respond:

- If the leukemia does not respond to any treatment, care focuses on supportive and palliative therapies to maintain quality of life.

HOW IS BCR::ABL1-POSITIVE B-ALL MANAGED?

BCR::ABL1-positive ALL is a rare but high-risk form of acute lymphoblastic leukemia. It occurs due to a Philadelphia chromosome abnormality, which creates the BCR::ABL1 fusion gene. This gene drives leukemia growth. The introduction of tyrosine kinase inhibitors (TKIs), such as imatinib, dasatinib, ponatinib etc. has greatly improved outcomes for these patients.

Front-Line Management

1. Treatment Approach:
   - Patients are treated with **intensive chemotherapy combined with a TKI** (like imatinib or dasatinib). It is important to note that the chemotherapy protocols for these patients are not different from those used for patients without BCR::ABL1 fusion gene.
   - TKIs block the BCR::ABL1 protein, which helps control the leukemia.

2. Key Trials and Results:
   - COG AALL0031:
   - Continuous use of imatinib during chemotherapy significantly improved survival (3-year EFS: 80.5% vs. historical 35%).
   - COG AALL0622:

- Dasatinib (a stronger TKI) showed similar survival outcomes to imatinib when combined with chemotherapy.
    - 5-year overall survival was 86%.
- EsPhALL Study:
    - Adding imatinib to chemotherapy improved 4-year survival compared to chemotherapy alone.
- St. Jude Total Therapy:
    - Adding TKIs (imatinib or dasatinib) reduced leukemia levels (MRD) and improved outcomes compared to pre-TKI treatment.

3. Emerging Strategies:
- Blinatumomab (an immunotherapy) and newer approaches like TKIs + Blinatumomab or Ponatinib + Blinatumomab are being tested for better results.
- These combinations may reduce the need for intensive chemotherapy.

4. Role of Stem Cell Transplant (HCT):
- In the past, HCT was standard for BCR::ABL1-positive ALL.
- Newer studies show that some patients who achieve remission with chemotherapy and TKIs may not need HCT, especially if MRD is negative.
- However, HCT remains an important option for high-risk patients or those with persistent disease.

Guidelines

For children and young adults (AYA) with BCR::ABL1-positive ALL:

1. Clinical Trials Preferred:
   - When possible, patients should be treated in a clinical trial.

2. Standard Treatment (if no trial is available):
   - Patients are treated with intensive chemotherapy combined with a TKI.
   - Response assessment is performed to determine the next steps:
     - Standard-Risk Patients (MRD-negative):
       - Continue with consolidation chemotherapy and maintenance therapy that includes a TKI.
       - Blinatumomab may be added during the post-remission phase based on recent data.
       - In some cases, stem cell transplant (HCT) may be considered as an alternative to maintenance therapy.
     - High-Risk Patients (less than CR after induction or MRD-positive at end of consolidation):
       - Options include:
         - Blinatumomab plus a TKI.
         - Tisagenlecleucel (CAR T-cell therapy) – preferably within a clinical trial.
       - Stem cell transplant (HCT) is recommended for these high-risk patients.
       - Post-transplant TKI therapy is advised to help prevent relapse.

3. Key Note About HCT:
   - HCT is not routinely needed for patients in first remission (CR1) if they achieve MRD negativity

(<0.01%) after consolidation and are on a strong pediatric chemotherapy regimen combined with a TKI.

Management of Relapsed or Refractory (R/R) Disease

Relapsed or refractory (R/R) BCR::ABL1-positive ALL is challenging, often due to resistance to TKIs. However, newer therapies are improving outcomes.

1. Chemotherapy + Tyrosine Kinase Inhibitors
- Imatinib and Dasatinib: Both TKIs have shown good response rates in relapsed disease.
- Ponatinib: Effective for patients resistant to imatinib or dasatinib, especially those with mutations like T315I.

2. Immunotherapy
- Blinatumomab:
  - An immunotherapy that targets CD19 and engages T cells to kill leukemia cells.
  - In adults with R/R BCR::ABL1-positive ALL, 36% achieved remission after blinatumomab treatment.
  - Blinatumomab can be combined with TKIs to improve outcomes.

3. CAR T-Cell Therapy
- CAR T cells are customized immune cells that target leukemia cells.
- Studies have shown high remission rates in patients with R/R ALL, including BCR::ABL1-

positive disease.
- Some patients can achieve long-term remission without needing a transplant after CAR T-cell therapy.

4. Inotuzumab Ozogamicin (InO)
- InO is a targeted therapy that delivers chemotherapy directly to leukemia cells carrying CD22.
- It has been effective in relapsed patients and is now approved for use in pediatric and adult patients.

5. Hematopoietic Cell Transplant (HCT)
- For patients with early relapse, HCT remains the most reliable option for a cure.
- A second transplant may be considered for those who relapse after their first HCT.

Guidelines

For patients whose leukemia comes back (relapsed) or does not respond to treatment (refractory):

1. General Approach:
   - Treatment is similar to R/R BCR::ABL1-negative ALL, but with the addition of TKIs.
   - Testing for BCR::ABL1 mutations (like the T315I mutation) is recommended to guide TKI selection.

2. TKI Options:
   - Dasatinib or imatinib are commonly used.
   - Ponatinib may be considered for resistant cases or specific mutations.

3. Additional Therapies:
 - Blinatumomab (an immunotherapy targeting CD19).
 - Tisagenlecleucel (CAR T-cell therapy), especially for patients who are not candidates for transplant.
 - HCT remains a key treatment option, especially for patients who respond to therapy but remain high risk.

MANAGEMENT OF T-ALL

Front-Line Management of T-ALL

T-ALL is treated with intense multiagent chemotherapy that aims to clear the leukemia early and prevent relapse. Treatment is based on results from key clinical trials:

1. COG AALL0434 Trial:
   - Nelarabine: Adding nelarabine (a chemotherapy drug) to treatment significantly improved outcomes for patients with high-risk T-ALL.
     - 4-Year Disease-Free Survival (DFS):
       - With nelarabine: 89%.
       - Without nelarabine: 83%.
     - Nelarabine was well-tolerated, with no significant added side effects like nerve or brain toxicity.
   - Methotrexate Intensification:
     - Capizzi MTX (a method of escalating doses) was better than high-dose methotrexate (HD-MTX) for preventing relapse.

2. COG AALL1231 Trial:
   - Bortezomib: Adding the drug bortezomib to chemotherapy improved outcomes for patients with T-cell lymphoblastic lymphoma (T-LL) but not T-ALL.

- Results also showed that cranial radiation (to prevent brain relapse) could be safely reduced without impacting outcomes.

3. DFCI Protocols 05-001 and 11-001:
 - Children with T-ALL treated with intensive protocols had good survival outcomes:
   - 5-Year Event-Free Survival (EFS): 81%.
   - 5-Year Overall Survival (OS): 90%.
 - Minimal Residual Disease (MRD) testing after early treatment is critical for identifying patients at higher risk of relapse.

4. Role of Stem Cell Transplant (HCT):
 - For T-ALL patients with positive MRD after initial treatment, HCT is recommended as part of their therapy to improve long-term outcomes.

Guidelines

- Treatment:
 - Pediatric and young adult (AYA) patients with T-ALL should ideally enroll in a clinical trial for the most advanced care options.
 - If a trial is not available, standard treatment is intensive chemotherapy.

- Risk Groups:
 After initial treatment (induction), patients are assessed to determine their risk level based on minimal residual disease (MRD) and other features:
 - Standard Risk:

- MRD <0.01% at day 29 (end of induction).
- No signs of CNS disease or testicular involvement.
- No steroid pretreatment before diagnosis.
- High Risk:
- Patients without standard-risk or very-high-risk features.
- Very High Risk:
- MRD >0.1% at the end of consolidation (later phase of treatment).

- Treatment for High and Very High Risk:
- Patients with very-high-risk disease may need alternative therapies and stem cell transplant (HCT) as part of their treatment.
- It is essential to reduce the disease burden (achieve MRD negativity) before proceeding to HCT.

Relapsed or Refractory (R/R) T-ALL Management

When T-ALL does not respond to treatment or comes back (relapse), achieving remission again is challenging. Available treatments include:

1. Nelarabine:
  - Approved for R/R T-ALL after at least two prior regimens.
  - About 55% of patients in first relapse respond to nelarabine.
  - Main side effect: Possible nerve-related toxicity.

2. Combination Regimens:
 - Nelarabine + Chemotherapy (like etoposide and cyclophosphamide): Increases response rates in relapsed disease.
 - Bortezomib-Based Regimens: Effective in some cases, as shown in the COG AALL07P1 study.

3. Venetoclax-Based Regimens:
 - Venetoclax combined with chemotherapy has shown promising results, especially in early T-cell precursor (ETP) ALL.

4. Daratumumab:
 - A monoclonal antibody targeting CD38, combined with chemotherapy, achieved good responses in clinical trials.

5. Hematopoietic Cell Transplant (HCT):
 - HCT remains the only curative option for relapsed or refractory T-ALL.
 - Achieving remission before transplant is critical.

Guidelines

- First Relapse:
 - Treatment starts with chemotherapy or participation in a clinical trial to achieve a second remission (CR2).
 - If remission is achieved:
 - Consolidation therapy continues with chemotherapy.
 - HCT is recommended for long-term remission.

- Multiple Relapses or Disease That Does Not Respond:

  - If the disease does not respond to therapy or relapses again, options include:
    - More chemotherapy to attempt remission.
    - Stem cell transplant (HCT) if remission is achieved.
  - If the disease does not respond to any treatment:
    - Supportive and palliative care to maintain quality of life is considered.

MANAGEMENT OF INFANT ALL

Front-Line Management of Infant ALL

Infant ALL (<12 months) often presents with aggressive features, including high WBC counts, CNS involvement, and KMT2A rearrangements. Treatment is intense but must balance efficacy with minimizing treatment-related toxicity.

Key Trials and Findings:

1. Interfant-99:
    - Used a hybrid regimen combining ALL and AML elements.
    - 4-year EFS: 47%; CR achieved in 94% of patients.
    - Poor prognostic factors:
        - Age <6 months
        - Poor prednisone response
        - High WBC count
        - KMT2A rearrangements

2. Interfant-06:
    - Compared lymphoid-style versus myeloid-style chemotherapy for consolidation.
    - Results: No overall benefit for myeloid-style therapy.
    - MRD-driven outcomes:
        - High MRD: Myeloid consolidation improved

DFS.
 - Low MRD: Lymphoid consolidation favored.
- Blinatumomab was added to Interfant-06 in a phase II study:
 - 2-year DFS: 81.6% (improved over standard therapy).
 - MRD negativity achieved more frequently with blinatumomab.

3. COG AALL0631:
- Added FLT3 inhibitor (lestaurtinib) to chemotherapy for KMT2A-rearranged ALL.
- Modified Interfant-99 induction was safer and improved CR rates.
- No benefit observed with lestaurtinib.

4. MLL-10 Trial (JPLSG):
- Stratified infants into low, intermediate, and high-risk groups.
- High-dose cytarabine intensification was used for KMT2A rearranged cases.
 - 3-year EFS:
   - Low-risk: 93.3%
   - Intermediate-risk: 94.4%
   - High-risk: 56.6%

Role of Hematopoietic Cell Transplant (HCT):
- The benefit of HCT in infant ALL remains unclear.
- Data from Interfant-99 suggested a role for HCT in high-risk KMT2A-rearranged ALL patients with:
 - Age <6 months
 - High WBC count

- Poor response to steroids

Guidelines

1. Clinical Trials Are Best:
 - Whenever possible, infants with ALL should be treated as part of a clinical trial. Clinical trials are carefully designed to test the most advanced and effective treatments available.

2. KMT2A Status Testing:
 - Doctors will test for KMT2A rearrangements, a common genetic change in infant ALL that affects treatment decisions.

3. Treatment Based on Risk Groups:
 - Standard Risk (KMT2A not rearranged):
 - Infants receive a treatment plan called Interfant-based chemotherapy (a mix of medications designed for infant ALL).
 - If no leukemia is detected after initial treatment (MRD-negative), the baby will continue risk-stratified chemotherapy.
 - If MRD (Minimal Residual Disease) is still present, treatment is made more intense to clear out the remaining cancer cells.
 - A newer medication, Blinatumomab, may also be added to improve outcomes.

 - High Risk (KMT2A rearranged):
 - Infants younger than 3 months, or babies under 6 months with very high white blood cell

counts (≥300,000), are treated more aggressively.

- Doctors may consider a stem cell transplant (HCT) to improve the chances of a cure, especially if there's still MRD after treatment.

- Transplant is safest if the baby is at least 6 months old and uses a method that avoids total body radiation (TBI).

- Intermediate Risk (KMT2A rearranged but no high-risk features):

- These infants are treated with maintenance chemotherapy to keep the leukemia from returning.

Management of Relapsed or Refractory (R/R) Infant ALL

- Outcomes for relapsed infant ALL are poor.
- Strategies used in R/R B-ALL and T-ALL apply here, including:
    - Blinatumomab
    - CAR T-cell therapy
    - Venetoclax-based regimens
    - HCT when remission is achieved

EVALUATION AND TREATMENT OF EXTRAMEDULLARY DISEASE

In ALL, leukemia cells sometimes spread outside the bone marrow to places like the brain and spinal fluid (CNS) or the testicles. This is called extramedullary disease, and it needs special treatment.

CNS Disease: Leukemia in the Brain and Spinal Fluid

1. What is CNS Involvement?
   - CNS leukemia happens when leukemia cells are found in the fluid around the brain and spinal cord. It is classified into three levels:
      - CNS-1: No leukemia cells in spinal fluid.
      - CNS-2: A small number of leukemia cells (WBC <5) in spinal fluid.
      - CNS-3: A high number of leukemia cells (WBC ≥5) or clinical symptoms like nerve palsy, seizures, or eye problems.
   - If the spinal tap is "traumatic" (accidentally mixes blood into the spinal fluid), doctors use the Steinherz-Bleyer formula to clarify the CNS status.

2. Why is Treating CNS Disease Important?
   - Without treatment, over 50% of patients will eventually develop CNS leukemia.
   - CNS involvement at diagnosis is linked to lower survival rates.

3. How is CNS Disease Treated?

- Intrathecal (IT) chemotherapy: Direct injection of chemotherapy (like methotrexate, cytarabine, or steroids) into the spinal fluid.
- Systemic chemotherapy: High doses of medications like methotrexate, cytarabine, and asparaginase.
- Cranial irradiation (radiation therapy to the brain): This is used only in very high-risk cases (CNS-3) because of long-term side effects, including learning problems, hormone issues, and risk of secondary cancers.

4. Is Radiation Always Needed?

- No. Advances in chemotherapy allow most patients to avoid radiation. Studies show that with intensive chemotherapy, the risk of CNS relapse can be reduced to around 3-5%.
- For patients who do need cranial radiation:
  - The standard dose is 18 Gy given in small daily doses.
  - It covers the whole brain and the back half of the eyes.

5. Long-Term Follow-Up After CNS Treatment:

- Patients treated with cranial radiation should be monitored for:
  - Learning delays or academic problems
  - Hormone changes (neuroendocrine issues)
  - Cataracts and vision problems
  - Risk of secondary cancers

Testicular Involvement: Leukemia in the Testes

1. What Happens if Leukemia is Found in the Testes?
   - In some boys, leukemia cells spread to the testes. If it doesn't resolve after initial chemotherapy, additional treatment is needed.

2. How is Testicular Disease Treated?
   - Radiation therapy to both testes is used. The total radiation dose is 24 Gy (delivered in small doses over time).

RESPONSE ASSESSMENT AND SURVEILLANCE

How Doctors Check Response to Treatment

Bone Marrow and Blood Tests

1. Complete Remission (CR):
   - No leukemia cells (blasts) in the blood.
   - No signs of leukemia outside the bone marrow (no enlarged lymph nodes, spleen, skin lumps, testicular masses, or CNS involvement).
   - Bone marrow tests must show <5% blasts (or <1% blasts using sensitive tests like flow cytometry or molecular testing).
   - Blood counts:
     - Neutrophils > 1000 cells/µL (to help fight infections).
     - Platelets > 100,000 cells/µL (to help blood clot).
   - Staying in remission for at least 4 weeks confirms CR.

2. CR with incomplete blood recovery (CRi):
   - Criteria for CR are met, but either:
     - Neutrophils stay <1000 cells/µL, or
     - Platelets remain <100,000 cells/µL.

3. Other Terms:
   - Refractory disease: Treatment did not result in CR after the first phase of therapy.

- Progressive disease (PD): Increase in leukemia cells in the blood, bone marrow, or development of new disease elsewhere.

- Relapsed disease: Leukemia cells reappear in the blood, bone marrow (>5%), or in other areas (like the brain) after CR was achieved.

CNS (Brain and Spinal Fluid) Disease

1. Remission in CNS Disease:
   - No leukemia cells in the spinal fluid (CNS-1).

2. CNS Relapse:
   - Return of CNS-3 status (≥5 white blood cells with leukemia cells in spinal fluid) or clinical signs of CNS leukemia (like nerve problems or brain involvement).
   - Two consecutive CNS-2 results (low-level leukemia cells in spinal fluid) may also signal relapse.

After Treatment: Monitoring and Surveillance

Once treatment (including maintenance therapy) is complete, regular follow-up visits are essential to monitor for any signs of relapse and assess overall health.

1. Physical Exams and Blood Tests:
   - First Year: Every 1–4 months.
   - Second Year: Every 2–6 months.
   - Third Year (and beyond): Every 6–12 months.

- These exams include:
  - Full physical exam (including a testicular exam for boys, if needed).
  - Blood tests (CBC with differential) to check for signs of relapse.
  - Liver function tests (until normal).

2. Bone Marrow and Spinal Fluid Tests:
- These are done only if relapse is suspected. Additional tests may include:
  - Flow cytometry (a sensitive test to detect leukemia cells).
  - Cytogenetics, molecular testing, and MRD testing.

3. Special Testing for BCR::ABL1-positive ALL:
- Regular checks of the BCR::ABL1 gene levels in the blood to monitor for relapse.

Monitoring for Late Effects

Survivors of ALL are monitored for long-term effects of treatment, including:

1. Heart Problems:
- Chemotherapy drugs like anthracyclines can affect the heart.
- An echocardiogram (heart ultrasound) is done regularly to check heart health.

2. Neurocognitive Effects:
- ALL treatments can cause learning or memory difficulties.

- Neuropsychological testing may be recommended if there are concerns.

3. Healthy Weight:
- Survivors are at higher risk for obesity. Maintaining a healthy diet, staying active, and making good lifestyle choices are essential.

4. Other Late Effects:
- Regular monitoring for issues like growth delays, reproductive health concerns, and risks of secondary cancers.
- The Children's Oncology Group (COG) guidelines provide detailed recommendations to address these concerns for childhood cancer survivors.

Regular check-ups and tests help detect any signs of leukemia returning early and monitor overall health. By catching problems early, doctors can ensure survivors live long, healthy lives after ALL treatment.

SUPPORTIVE CARE FOR PEDIATRIC PATIENTS WITH ALL

Supportive care is essential to ensure children with ALL can safely tolerate intensive treatments and receive the best outcomes. Here's a simple breakdown of the key supportive care measures:

Infection Control

- Increased Risk for Infections: Chemotherapy weakens the immune system, making children more vulnerable to infections (bacterial, fungal, and viral).
- What's Done:
  - Antibiotics and Antifungals: Given as prevention (prophylaxis) throughout treatment.
  - Example: Trimethoprim/Sulfamethoxazole (TMP/SMX) for preventing lung infections caused by Pneumocystis jirovecii. Alternatives like atovaquone may be used if TMP/SMX isn't tolerated.
  - Broad-spectrum antibiotics: Started immediately if a fever develops, especially during neutropenia (low white blood cell counts).
  - Vaccines: Routine vaccines may be delayed, but inactivated vaccines can often be resumed 3 months after chemotherapy ends.

Managing Tumor Lysis Syndrome (TLS)

- TLS happens when chemotherapy quickly kills

leukemia cells, releasing their contents into the blood and causing kidney, heart, or nerve problems.
- What's Done:
 - IV Fluids: Hydration is essential to protect the kidneys.
 - Allopurinol or Rasburicase: Medicines help lower uric acid levels.

Methotrexate (MTX) Toxicity Management

- High doses of methotrexate can sometimes harm the kidneys, liver, or brain.
- What's Done:
 - Glucarpidase (a rescue medicine) is used to clear toxic levels of methotrexate from the body.
 - Leucovorin rescue is used alongside methotrexate to protect healthy cells.
 - Seizures or stroke-like symptoms: These side effects may resolve on their own, but anti-seizure medicines may be used temporarily.

Cardiotoxicity (Heart Problems) with Anthracyclines

- Chemotherapy drugs like doxorubicin can damage the heart.
- What's Done:
 - Dexrazoxane: A medicine given with chemotherapy to protect the heart.
 - Heart check-ups (echocardiograms): Regular tests to monitor heart health.

Steroid-Related Side Effects

- Short-Term Side Effects:
  - High blood sugar: Blood sugar monitoring and a healthy diet help prevent complications.
  - Muscle weakness, mood changes, ulcers, or acid reflux: Medications like antacids can help manage stomach issues.
- Long-Term Side Effects:
  - Bone damage (osteonecrosis): This often affects the hips and knees, especially in teens. MRI scans can check for bone damage.
  - Prevention: Adjustments to steroids or switching from dexamethasone to prednisone may help.

Vincristine-Related Nerve Damage

- Nerve Issues: Vincristine can cause nerve pain, constipation, and muscle weakness.
- What's Done:
  - Adjust the dose if severe symptoms occur.
  - Use medications like gabapentin for nerve pain.
  - Prevent constipation with laxatives and proper diet.

Asparaginase Toxicity Management

- Common Issues: Allergic reactions, pancreatitis (severe abdominal pain), blood clotting issues, or liver problems.
- What's Done:
  - Children are closely monitored during and after asparaginase treatment.
  - Alternatives or adjustments to treatment may be

used if severe side effects occur.

Pain Management

- Bone Pain: Common with chemotherapy and steroids.
- Nerve Pain: Seen with vincristine treatment.
- What's Done:
  - Pain-relief medicines like acetaminophen, gabapentin, or opioids may be used when needed.
  - Consultation with pediatric pain specialists if severe pain persists.

Nutritional Support

- What's Done:
  - Nutritional support: For weight loss, options include appetite stimulants or feeding tubes (if needed).
  - Encourage physical activity to maintain muscle strength and prevent weight gain.

Psychological and Cognitive Support

- Children with ALL may experience:
  - Learning or memory difficulties due to chemotherapy.
  - Emotional or mood changes related to steroids or treatment.
- What's Done:
  - Regular neuropsychological tests to monitor learning and development.
  - Counseling or therapy to address emotional challenges.

Blood Transfusions

- Blood or platelet transfusions are often needed for low blood counts.
- Special care is taken to use safe, irradiated blood products to avoid complications.

Supportive care focuses on preventing and managing treatment side effects so children can safely complete therapy. Regular monitoring, timely interventions, and a tailored approach for each patient ensure the best possible care and long-term outcomes.

WHAT IS THE TYPICAL EXPERIENCE OF A PATIENT WITH ALL AND THEIR FAMILY DURING THE COURSE OF DIAGNOSIS AND TREATMENT?

A diagnosis of ALL is life-changing for both the patient and their family. It involves physical, emotional, financial, and social challenges throughout the intensive, multi-phase treatment journey, often lasting 2-3 years.

1. Emotional Impact of Diagnosis

For the Family:
- Shock and Denial: Families often experience disbelief when they hear the word "cancer."
- Fear and Anxiety: Concerns about survival, treatment effectiveness, and how the child will cope dominate their thoughts.
- Guilt: Parents may question whether they missed early symptoms or contributed to the disease in some way.
- Loss of Normalcy: The diagnosis disrupts school, work, and everyday routines.
- Uncertainty: Families face constant worry about relapses, treatment side effects, and long-term outcomes.

For the Patient:
- Fear of the Unknown: Young children often do not understand the disease but fear hospital stays,

needles, and tests.

- Isolation: Prolonged hospital stays can be lonely, as the child is separated from friends, school, and siblings.
- Body Changes: Hair loss, weight gain (steroids), or weakness due to treatment can affect self-esteem in older children and teenagers.
- Mood Swings: Steroids can cause significant emotional outbursts and changes in behavior.

2. The Physical Journey

A. Phases of Treatment

ALL treatment involves multiple phases: induction, consolidation/intensification, and maintenance therapy. Each phase comes with its own challenges.

- Induction (4-6 weeks): The goal is to eliminate leukemia cells and achieve remission.
    - Frequent lumbar punctures for CNS-directed therapy.
    - Continuous monitoring of blood counts and response to treatment.
    - Hospital admissions are common due to infection risk or severe side effects.

- Consolidation/Intensification (Several months): This phase targets remaining leukemia cells to prevent relapse.
    - Intensive chemotherapy schedules.
    - Frequent visits to the hospital for chemotherapy infusions and monitoring.

- Maintenance (1.5–2 years): Long-term, less-intensive chemotherapy to keep leukemia in remission.
    - Oral medications at home and periodic hospital visits.
    - Balance between treatment and returning to "normal" life like school and activities.

B. Side Effects of Chemotherapy

Patients endure various physical side effects during treatment, including:
- Fatigue: Extreme tiredness limits physical activity and social engagement.
- Nausea and Vomiting: Chemotherapy causes gastrointestinal upset, requiring antiemetics.
- Hair Loss: A visible and often emotional side effect.
- Infections: Chemotherapy weakens the immune system, leading to high infection risks.
- Mouth Sores and Pain: Mucositis can make eating and talking difficult.
- Bone Pain and Neuropathy: Drugs like steroids and vincristine can cause severe pain or nerve damage.
- Weight Changes:
    - Weight Gain: Steroids increase appetite, leading to rapid weight gain.
    - Weight Loss: Appetite suppression, nausea, or mouth sores may cause malnutrition.
- Bleeding and Bruising: Low platelet counts increase the risk of bleeding.
- Liver and Kidney Issues: Chemotherapy toxicity can cause organ damage.

- Cognitive Issues: Memory and focus can be impacted, especially after CNS-directed therapy.

3. Hospital Experience

- Frequent Visits and Stays:
    - Many hospital visits for chemotherapy, blood tests, imaging scans, lumbar punctures, and bone marrow aspirations.
    - Prolonged admissions for infections, side effects, or complications.

- Needle Sticks and Procedures:
    - Port or Central Line: A surgically implanted catheter allows for blood draws and chemotherapy, reducing needle sticks but requiring proper care.
    - Frequent lumbar punctures for chemotherapy into the spinal fluid.

- Isolation Precautions:
    - Patients with low immunity may need to stay in isolation to avoid infections, which is particularly hard for young children.

4. Financial and Practical Challenges

- Medical Costs: Even with insurance, families face significant expenses, including hospital stays, medications, and supportive care.
- Time Off Work: Parents often take unpaid leave or quit their jobs to care for the child.
- Travel Costs: Frequent trips to treatment centers add transportation, lodging, and meal expenses.
- Managing Siblings: Siblings may feel neglected, as

parents spend time at the hospital.

5. Social Disruption

- School Absences:
    - The child misses school due to treatment and hospitalization.
    - Returning to school can be challenging due to fatigue, immune suppression, or cognitive effects.
- Limited Social Interaction:
    - Infections prevent attendance at birthday parties, gatherings, or events.
    - Friends may not understand the illness or its limitations.
- Stigma and Isolation:
    - Parents may feel isolated from their community and support system.
    - Older children and teens struggle with feelings of being "different."

6. Long-Term Effects and Surveillance

- Physical:
    - Growth delays, endocrine issues, heart or kidney damage, or bone damage (osteonecrosis).
    - Fertility concerns due to chemotherapy exposure.
- Neurocognitive Issues:
    - Problems with memory, attention, and learning may arise, impacting school performance.
- Emotional and Psychological Impact:
    - Anxiety and fear of relapse.
    - Depression or PTSD in parents and older

patients.
- Survivors often need ongoing counseling to process their experiences.
- Monitoring for Late Effects:
- Long-term medical follow-ups include heart tests, neuropsychological assessments, and cancer screenings to detect secondary malignancies.

7. Supportive Care

- Pain Management: Medications for bone pain, neuropathy, and general discomfort.
- Nutritional Support: Proper diet or feeding support to prevent weight loss or malnutrition.
- Counseling and Psychosocial Support: Therapy helps families and patients cope with stress, grief, and anxiety.
- Support Groups: Connecting with other families going through similar experiences provides emotional support.

The journey through ALL is undeniably challenging, but many families discover unexpected sources of strength and hope along the way. For many, the experience brings families closer as they face the illness together. "We learned to lean on each other like never before," one parent shared. These trials often forge deeper bonds, creating a sense of unity and mutual support.

Children undergoing treatment frequently display extraordinary resilience and courage. "My child's bravery amazed me every day," a mother recalled.

Their determination often inspires not just their families but also their caregivers and communities.

The experience also brings a new perspective on life. Families learn to appreciate life's small joys—moments that might have otherwise gone unnoticed. "We started celebrating the little victories, like a good blood count or a day without pain," one father explained.

Support from friends, extended family, charities, and the broader community plays a vital role during this time. Whether it's emotional encouragement, financial assistance, or simply being present, this network becomes a pillar of strength. "We felt surrounded by kindness, even from people we barely knew," another family shared.

While the journey through ALL is fraught with difficulty, these moments of connection, courage, and support often provide a profound sense of hope and resilience.

WHAT LIFESTYLE ADVICE, FOOD PREFERENCES, AND PRECAUTIONS SHOULD BE FOLLOWED BY PATIENTS UNDERGOING ALL TREATMENT?

During treatment for ALL, it's essential to balance medical care with supportive lifestyle practices. Proper nutrition, physical activity, precautions to prevent infections, and emotional well-being all play key roles in improving treatment outcomes and quality of life.

1. Nutrition and Food Preferences

Chemotherapy and ALL treatment can affect appetite, digestion, and taste preferences. The goal is to provide adequate calories, protein, and essential nutrients to:
- Support the immune system.
- Maintain energy levels.
- Aid recovery and tissue repair.

Food Recommendations:
- High-Protein Foods: Protein is essential for growth, repair, and fighting infections. Include:
  - Eggs, fish, chicken, lean meats.
  - Paneer, tofu, lentils, chickpeas, beans.
  - Nuts, seeds, and nut butters (almond butter, peanut butter).
  - Dairy products like yogurt, milk, and cheese.

- Easily Digestible Carbs:
  - Rice, pasta, potatoes, oats, quinoa.
  - Whole wheat bread (if tolerated).
  - Bananas, applesauce, boiled vegetables.

- Healthy Fats: To provide energy and promote weight gain:
  - Avocados, olive oil, ghee (in moderation).
  - Nuts and seeds.
  - Fatty fish (salmon, mackerel) for omega-3 fatty acids.

- Fruits and Vegetables:
  - Include cooked fruits and vegetables to minimize infection risk.
  - Avoid raw or unwashed produce; peeling fruit is safer.
  - Carrots, sweet potatoes, spinach, and berries (when cooked) provide antioxidants.

- Hydration:
  - Drink plenty of fluids to avoid dehydration, especially during chemotherapy.
  - Water, coconut water, soups, fresh homemade juice, and oral rehydration solutions (ORS) are ideal.

Tips for Loss of Appetite or Taste Changes:
- Offer small, frequent meals rather than large portions.
- Serve foods at room temperature to reduce strong odors.
- Encourage favorite meals, even if repetitive.

- Try smoothies, milkshakes, or soups if chewing is difficult.
- Add flavor with herbs, lemon juice, or mild spices.

Avoid:
- Raw or undercooked meat, fish, eggs, and unpasteurized dairy (infection risk).
- Street food or food prepared in unhygienic conditions.
- Sugary, processed, or fried foods in excess.
- Artificial sweeteners or supplements without doctor approval.

2. Infection Prevention

ALL treatment suppresses the immune system, increasing the risk of infections. Taking precautions is critical:

- Hygiene Practices:
  - Wash hands frequently with soap and water (patients and caregivers).
  - Use alcohol-based hand sanitizers when soap is unavailable.
  - Practice good oral hygiene: gentle tooth brushing, rinsing after meals.

- Environment:
  - Avoid crowded places, malls, and public transport during peak seasons (flu, COVID-19).
  - Ensure the patient's living space is clean, dust-free, and well-ventilated.
  - Avoid gardening or contact with soil (risk of

fungal infections).

- Food Safety:
  - Wash fruits and vegetables thoroughly.
  - Cook all meats and eggs fully.
  - Avoid stale or leftover food.

- Personal Items:
  - Use a separate toothbrush, towels, and utensils for the patient.
  - Replace toothbrushes regularly.

- Vaccination:
  - Avoid live vaccines during treatment. Consult with the oncologist regarding vaccination schedules (e.g., flu shots).

- Pets:
  - Avoid close contact with pets' saliva or feces.
  - Keep pets clean and well-groomed.

- Mask Usage:
  - Wear a mask in hospital settings or around sick individuals.

3. Physical Activity and Rest

- Exercise:
  - Light activity, such as walking or gentle yoga, helps improve energy levels, reduce fatigue, and enhance mood.
  - Avoid strenuous or risky activities, especially during periods of low blood counts.

- Rest and Sleep:
  - Encourage 8-10 hours of sleep per night with daytime naps if needed.
  - Create a quiet, calming environment for rest.
  - Practice relaxation techniques like deep breathing or meditation.

4. Emotional Well-being

- For the Patient:
  - Engage in Fun Activities: Reading, art, music, board games, or watching favorite shows can distract and lift spirits.
  - Maintain Social Connections: Virtual or in-person chats with friends can help reduce isolation.
  - Counseling and Support Groups: For older children or teenagers, counseling helps manage anxiety, sadness, or fear.

- For the Family:
  - Seek Support: Family members can benefit from therapy or peer support groups to share experiences.
  - Stay Informed: Understanding the treatment plan helps reduce anxiety.
  - Set a Routine: Maintaining some structure, even during treatment, can improve well-being.

5. School and Daily Activities

- School Continuity:
  - Encourage schoolwork during maintenance therapy or hospital stays when energy permits.
  - Work with teachers for accommodations (home-

based learning, flexible deadlines).

- Routines:
  - Structure the day with time for meals, rest, light activity, and fun.
  - Be flexible on tough days, and prioritize the patient's comfort.

6. Precautions with Specific Treatments

- Steroids:
  - Monitor for mood changes and irritability.
  - Manage weight gain by encouraging healthy snacks and meals.
  - Check blood sugar levels for steroid-induced hyperglycemia.

- Vincristine (Neuropathy):
  - Watch for muscle weakness or pain. Encourage gentle stretching exercises.

- Asparaginase (Pancreatitis Risk):
  - Report any abdominal pain, nausea, or vomiting immediately.

- Methotrexate (Neurotoxicity):
  - Look for stroke-like symptoms or seizures; seek immediate care.

7. Long-term Health and Wellness

- Nutrition: Maintain a balanced, nutrient-dense diet to help with recovery and growth post-treatment.

- Exercise: Encourage regular physical activity to rebuild strength and prevent obesity.
- Follow-ups: Regular medical checkups are essential for detecting relapses or late side effects (cardiac, bone, or endocrine issues).
- Healthy Lifestyle: Promote a non-smoking, drug-free, and alcohol-free lifestyle for long-term health.

WHAT ARE THE COMMON COMPLICATIONS OF ALL TREATMENT, AND HOW CAN FAMILIES EFFECTIVELY MANAGE THEM?

During treatment for ALL, patients may face several complications due to the disease itself, chemotherapy, or prolonged immunosuppression. Below are key complications, their signs/symptoms, and strategies for family members to help manage them effectively.

1. Infections

Why It Happens:
- Chemotherapy weakens the immune system, making the patient prone to bacterial, viral, and fungal infections.

Signs to Watch For:
- Fever (temperature ≥100.4°F or 38°C).
- Cough, sore throat, or difficulty breathing.
- Diarrhea, vomiting, or abdominal pain.
- Skin rashes, redness, or swelling.
- Mouth sores or white patches in the mouth (fungal infection).

Family Management Tips:
- Immediate Action for Fever: Report fever to the treating doctor immediately; antibiotics may be needed.
- Strict Hygiene:
  - Frequent handwashing for the patient and family.

- Clean toys, utensils, and living areas daily.
- Avoid Infection Sources:
  - Keep the patient away from sick individuals and crowded places.
  - Limit visitors and discourage physical contact (e.g., handshakes).
- Prophylaxis: Ensure the patient takes all prescribed antibacterial, antiviral, and antifungal medications.
- Monitor for Symptoms: Early intervention is critical for infections.

2. Bleeding and Bruising

Why It Happens:
- Low platelet counts due to chemotherapy cause easy bruising and bleeding.

Signs to Watch For:
- Easy bruising, tiny red spots on the skin (petechiae).
- Nosebleeds, gum bleeding, or prolonged bleeding from minor cuts.
- Blood in urine, stool, or vomit.
- Headache, dizziness, or vomiting, which may indicate internal bleeding.

Family Management Tips:
- Prevent Injuries:
  - Use soft toothbrushes and avoid flossing.
  - Trim nails short to prevent scratches.
  - Avoid contact sports or activities with a fall risk.
- Minimize Bleeding Risks:
  - Avoid sharp objects, hard foods, and rough

handling.
  - Use electric razors instead of blades.
- Monitor Symptoms: Report any signs of bleeding or bruising to the doctor immediately.
- Transfusions: Be prepared for platelet transfusions if recommended by the doctor.

3. Nausea and Vomiting
Why It Happens:
- Chemotherapy often triggers nausea and vomiting as a side effect.

Family Management Tips:
- Dietary Adjustments:
  - Offer bland, easily digestible foods like rice, toast, or applesauce.
  - Serve smaller, frequent meals rather than large portions.
  - Avoid greasy, spicy, or strong-smelling foods.
- Hydration:
  - Give small sips of water, ORS, or diluted juices.
  - Ice chips or popsicles can help.
- Medication Support: Ensure antiemetic medications are taken as prescribed.
- Timing: Offer meals when nausea is less severe (e.g., before chemotherapy or at non-peak hours).

4. Mouth Sores (Mucositis)
Why It Happens:
- Chemotherapy damages the lining of the mouth and throat, leading to painful sores.

Signs to Watch For:

- Painful mouth ulcers, difficulty eating or swallowing, and drooling.

Family Management Tips:
- Oral Hygiene:
  - Rinse the mouth frequently with saline or prescribed mouthwash.
  - Avoid alcohol-based mouthwashes, as they can worsen irritation.
- Pain Management:
  - Use prescribed pain-relief gels or medications.
- Diet Adjustments:
  - Serve soft, cold, or pureed foods like yogurt, smoothies, or mashed potatoes.
  - Avoid acidic, spicy, or rough foods that may worsen sores.

5. Bone Pain and Joint Pain

Why It Happens:
- Chemotherapy (especially steroids and vincristine) can cause bone and nerve pain.

Family Management Tips:
- Pain Management:
  - Give prescribed pain medications like paracetamol (avoid NSAIDs like ibuprofen unless advised).
  - Apply warm compresses to aching joints or muscles.
- Supportive Care:
  - Encourage gentle stretching or light activities to improve mobility.

- Avoid strenuous activities that may worsen the pain.
- Comfort: Ensure the child has a comfortable sleeping area with proper support.

6. Fatigue
Why It Happens:
- Chemotherapy, anemia, and the stress of treatment contribute to fatigue.

Family Management Tips:
- Encourage Rest:
  - Allow naps or breaks during the day.
  - Create a relaxing bedtime routine for quality sleep.
- Balanced Activity:
  - Encourage light activities like short walks or gentle yoga to improve energy levels.
- Nutrition and Hydration: Offer high-protein, high-calorie foods to maintain energy.

7. Steroid-Related Complications
Common Issues:
- Weight gain, mood swings, irritability, hyperglycemia, and risk of infection.

Family Management Tips:
- Diet:
  - Avoid high-sodium, sugary, and fried foods to manage weight gain.
  - Offer nutritious snacks like fruits, vegetables, and nuts.

- Mood Support:
  - Be patient with mood swings and irritability; encourage relaxation techniques.
  - Provide reassurance and emotional support.
- Monitor Blood Sugar: Check for increased thirst, frequent urination, or tiredness. Report these to the doctor.

8. Constipation and Neuropathy

Why It Happens:
- Chemotherapy drugs like vincristine can cause nerve damage and constipation.

Family Management Tips:
- Diet:
  - Increase fiber intake (oats, fruits, vegetables).
  - Encourage plenty of fluids.
- Physical Activity: Light movement can help bowel function.
- Medications: Give stool softeners or laxatives if prescribed.
- Neuropathy: Watch for numbness, tingling, or difficulty walking. Report symptoms promptly.

9. Emotional Stress and Anxiety

Why It Happens:
- The patient and family may experience anxiety, fear, and sadness due to treatment and its challenges.

Family Management Tips:
- Open Communication: Encourage the child to express their feelings and listen without judgment.

- Fun Activities: Engage in art, music, storytelling, or games to distract from stress.
- Support Groups: Connect with other families through hospital-organized groups.
- Counseling: Seek professional support for mental health when needed.

10. Weight Loss or Weight Gain
Family Management Tips:
- For Weight Loss:
   - Offer calorie-dense foods like smoothies, milkshakes, peanut butter, and cheese.
   - Small, frequent meals can help.
- For Weight Gain (Steroid-Induced):
   - Limit processed or sugary foods.
   - Focus on balanced meals with protein, healthy fats, and vegetables.

11. Long-term Side Effects
Post-treatment, patients may experience:
- Fatigue, bone health issues, or cognitive effects.
- Cardiac problems (from anthracyclines).

Family Role:
- Follow-ups: Ensure regular checkups to monitor for late effects.
- Healthy Lifestyle: Encourage physical activity, good nutrition, and hydration.
- Emotional Support: Continue counseling and mental health care.

ALL treatment is a challenging journey that requires vigilance and support from families. By watching for complications, maintaining a clean and safe environment, supporting nutrition and emotional health, and ensuring open communication with healthcare providers, families can help manage treatment side effects and improve their child's overall well-being.

LETTER TO A READER

Dearest Reader,

As we draw the curtain on this modest endeavor, let us reflect upon the resilience of the human spirit, which shines brightest in the face of adversity. The journey through ALL, though fraught with trials, is one of courage, perseverance, and hope—a testament to the strength of families united by love. Though the path may seem steep and shadowed at times, remember that even the darkest clouds may part to reveal a brighter horizon.

You, as parents and caregivers, have been endowed with a noble charge: to nurture, protect, and champion your child through this challenging chapter of their life. Let each step, no matter how small, be a triumph, and let each moment of joy, however fleeting, be a cherished treasure. Trust in the wisdom of those who guide you—the physicians, nurses, and countless others whose labor is rooted in compassion and knowledge.

And for you, young reader, should you find yourself in the throes of this tale, take heart. You are the hero of your story, endowed with strength beyond measure. Know that you are never alone, for the love of your family and the care of countless hands accompany you.

Thus, with a spirit of optimism and unshaken resolve, let us turn the page, confident that the future holds promise, healing, and the warm embrace of a life well-lived.

Yours most sincerely,
Dr. Bhratri Bhushan, MD, DM

ABOUT THE AUTHOR

Dr. Bhratri Bhushan

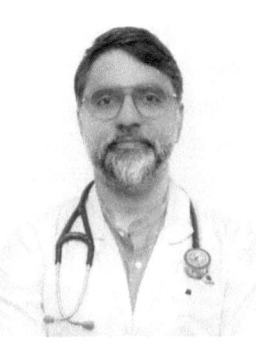

Dr. Bhratri Bhushan is a consultant medical oncologist and hematologist. He has a rich academic and research background, having published more than two hundred books on the subjects of oncology and internal medicine. His scholarly contributions have been featured in renowned journals of medical literature. For a comprehensive collection of his works, please visit his AuthorCentral page at www.amazon.com/author/bhratribhushan